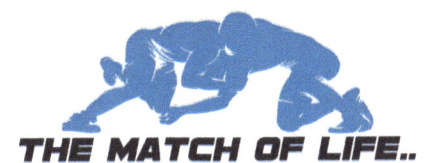

Presents...

POWER

OF

POSITIVE THINKING...

COPYRIGHT © 2019. ALL RIGHTS RESERVED.

No part of this publication may be reproduced, distributed, or transmitted in any form or by any means, including photocopying, recording, or other electronic or mechanical methods, or by any information storage and retrieval system without the prior written permission of the publisher, except in the case of very brief quotations embodied in critical reviews and certain other noncommercial uses permitted by copyright law.

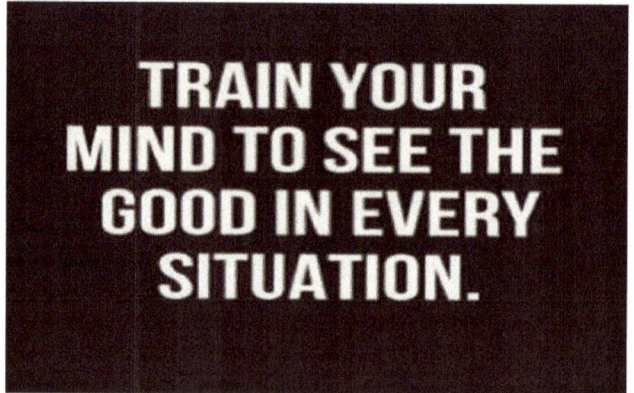

POWER OF POSITIVE THINKING.

People who are blessed with the quality to energize their thought process with mammoth degree of positivity are sure enough to achieve the success in all fronts in professional and social life. They are classified as people with a positive frame of mind and do not get provoked and indulge in any sort of mental block. They are also like many others; but only difference is that they do not delve much on their weaknesses and do not blame their luck for any failures. They consider the failures as a stepping stone which shows them the path of success. This is one side of the coin. The opposite side is also prevalent. That means there are people who always focus attention to their past mistakes, murmur, curse the environment and situations for failures. These thoughts make their minds distract from positivity and abundance of failures will always rattle their inner self.

You have to **remember** that you are always better than what you are. You have to have full trust on your ability and intelligence. Your body is like one of the highly acclaimed machines and your brain deserves to be a critical asset. You can definitely accept the challenges of the surroundings with all these combinations. To make these all happen, a personality trait which is a very important factor for anybody, to amplify - is known as **attitude**. This attitude helps you to induce the power of thinking in a very positive way and this eight letters word can create a magic wind for you. As per Winston Churchill, "An attitude is a small ingredient, but makes a lot of difference in your life."

1. **Power of thoughts:**

Any action is a reflection of thought process which is guided by a positive or a negative thought. You will become a successful person, when you are influenced by lifting up your thoughts. The research data shows that the working pattern of your body and your thoughts have interconnection. If you are endowed with a positive frame of mind and thoughts, you will be able to lift your spirit. Contrarily, if your mind is always hovered with the thoughts of failures, surely you would encounter the same only. In my professional life, I come across different types of personalities and I have the privilege to segregate the intellectual lot with haughty nature, and ample money power versus the lot with less materialistic power, but with intensive positive attitudinal perch of mind. And, to the best of the best of my knowledge, I opine that the second lot makes history and always smile in their lives beatifically.

You take the instance of the environment either of office or work, all your acts will be governed by thoughts. Depending on the gravity of your acts for any assignment, you will be able to judge your performance. The level of performance will enhance when the acts will be influenced by a positive attitude. You will be able to raise the output beyond the expected level because of the constructive behaviour and so consequence of the results therefore, will be always positive.

The success is not a derivative of any lose efforts. It is a structural and a continuous process of development of various skills and knowledge and when bestowed with positive thoughts, right actions are guaranteed to happen. So, for advancement in life, fill up your mind with positive, productive and enriching thoughts. This will ensure you for a noticeable difference in your attitude towards the life.

2. Sole searching:

Many a time, in your life, you feel yourself less enthusiastic and ponder on anxieties caused due to various perceptions which may or may not have any relationship with your career, social life or materialistic despondency. But, such behaviour is quite radical. Because, even otherwise your brilliancy is undoubtedly beyond questionable, the negative thoughts may crop up in your mind just because of above situations. Whatever the positive frame of mind you possess, negative thoughts as stated above, will destroy the energy of your inner self and you will be under shackles of despair. Please remember that nothing is achievable easily and so you have to toil excessively and endlessly to earn other peoples support services, their co-operation and good wishes

This is just a guide line, but to energize your inner self with the power of positive thought, you have to continuously introspect till the time; you recognize the truth of its importance.

3. Build up yourself:

A normal person of average caliber, even otherwise possesses several abilities which are up to the mark with respect to any prevailing standard may require to invest for his overall growth. You have to continuously upgrade your skills, knowledge, and keenness to float in the corporate jungle. Always concentrate on the job which you like and know more about the same. This keenness will only bring more colour to your life and your career graph will zoom.

4. Plan, follow and improve:

If your planning is perfect and accurate, the accomplishment of a job will be far above than the expected result. To do this, you have to be extremely effective to master the techniques of the job. You have to have enough skills to undertake the job. The role of planning, in this case, is a very important thing. If the planning is foolproof, the results cannot be haywire. A person, who does not recognize the importance of the planning, will be clueless and cannot reach to a desired destination. Here comes the perspective of the attitude. Without this personality trait, it is extremely difficult to achieve any success in the life. The success is like a war which is full of mirth and despondency. If your planning is strong enough and devised with scientific approaches, then the success cannot delude you.

It is very essential to dwell on the strengths in stead of the weaknesses. No one should sulk on what they do not have, rather a concentration of the entire focus is to be put forward what we have. The celebrities from all round the corner never brood in their limitations as their attitudinal behaviour will always guide them to the path of positive thinking. And this character alone will be benevolent for their success in their lives. Always keep an attitude to constantly upgrade yourself because there is no substitute for the same. By indulging for self development, you will be in a position to improve upon your performance in any field. No sooner, you will show complacent, downfall will start and you will not be in a position to filter further.

5. Attitude:

This can be spelt as follows:

A = Attribute - to be positive.

T = Try - to change if the attitude is negative

T = Total control - to negate your negative thoughts.

I = Instinct - to use to visualize the positive, even in adversity.

T = Think - to start every thing with positive and constructive approach.

U = Understand - all your inherent strengths.

D = Develop - your conscious to achieve the best.

E = Energize - your inner self to influence outer self to be always positive.

You have to remember that in a professional as well as social environment, your attitude will affect other people and what they think of you. In today's' competitive working environment, when you have to work in a team, your attitude is one of the main criteria for your success. Without a balanced attitude, it will be tricky for you to overcome the obstacles which are developed off and on. So, thoughts are to be sensitized and to be added with fantasies to eradicate the negative emotions. By practicing this hypothesis, gradually, mind will be energized to pursue the positive aspect of the thoughts. This will, in turn, become a habit and transform to the attitude.

6. Attitudinal behaviour and its impact on career:

This personality trait is very important determinant, at the start of your professional career, because when you appear for interview, the interviewers gauze subtly your this quality. Because, they know that they can train you to their job requirement, but it is extremely difficult for them to change your attitude.

You will be able to conquer any obstacles, if you have a positive attitude. This positive attitude will be able to blossom your inherent quality to focus your attention to the brighter side of any things.

In my professional career of marketing, as a departmental head since long, I always encourage on coaching of my people to take out the best possible output from them. I have noticed that if a person has a positive attitude and the ability of "can do confidence," he will, by and large, achieve the success even he is weak in some sphere of the knowledge. On the contrary, may be, some people are very brilliant but totally engrossed with a negative attitude, they are the maximum sufferers. In today's' global competitive arena, the companies are always in search of the people, who show the immense power of positive attitude in all spheres.

Mostly, all the companies are now conducting psychometric analytical tests to measure the candidates attitude and then conclude about the potentiality of the success of a candidate. Individually, they are capable to exhibit tremendous performance when they are blessed with the positive frame of mind. You have to become a master of the mind but not its slave. By doing this, you will be able to control your mind and will be in a position to always concentrate on positive things of the surroundings.

7. **Keep away from negative:**

The life is completely full of mysteries of successes and failures. Everyone has to face this naked truth. Failures doom the strengths of a person and develop negative consequences. Whatever they see, it will be full of darkness. The famous couplet of "Genesis" of the Bible says that during the creation of the universe, the first thing, God said "Let there be a light" because the total universe was under the clutch of the darkness. God never said, "Let there be darkness." In the similar way, in our day to day life, we have to always encounter the darkness with a light. If you are calm and quiet, and maintain a positive frame of mind even in your disastrous state of your life, a habit of positiveness will grow which will enable you to think always to see the brighter side of the life only. I would like to put forward a classic example of positive attitude which many of us know very well. Mr. Iswarchandra Vidyasagar, the eminent scholar, was summoned one day by her mother to meet. When he reached to the river Damodar during late evening, he could not find any boat because of heavy tidal conditions. But he had made up his mind to meet her mother by hook or by crook and so, he ignored the fanatic condition of the river. He swam and reached to his house late night to touch the feet of her mother. What a positive attitude he showed! This example glorifies, how to steer away the darkness and the negativity of the life.

8. Attitude -vs- Success:

An attitude and a success, both are hand in gloves. The success is directly proportional to the positive attitude. You can never dream a success without a positive attitude. "I can do" attitude only can plan your actions into reality and results. Please keep in mind that any success is not easily achievable. Mind boggling efforts, pain-staking work, eradication of negative thoughts, and tremendous perseverance are required to feel the stepping stone of success. In your this endeavour, you will come across resources crunch, negative criticism from peers and friends, hurdles of circumstances but keep your all positive thoughts intact for your motivation to perform the best and success will be guaranteed.

There is no magic wind for the success. It comes to you automatically, if you exert your best efforts with brimming confidence of mind. When you engage yourself in any purposeful action, maximize your potentialities, concentrate and focus all your attentions to the actions with constructive and positive thoughts, you will always find your missions completed.

As a marketing coach in my present employment, I impart training to the young engineers for their career upbringing. To make them aware of the fundamental principles of the products development versus marketing operations, I profusely teach them the importance of the attitude. During the initial six months of probation training, I ensure them to concentrate on positive thoughts, or else I make them understand that they will face enormous problems in achieving their career goals.

Further, many people think that positive thoughts are the domain of some particular persons. But, it is not correct. Even, if you are average qualified, have mediocre brain, and aged, you can always learn and practice the power of positive thoughts. To maintain the thought process in a positive direction, you need not be over qualified or have super brain power. It is only a matter of habit that how you shut the door of your mind and prevent the entry of any negative thoughts. This is the main and important quality which is required to sharpen the skill to think always positive. It is true that negative thoughts cannot be erased, but if you put layers after layers of positive thoughts into your mind, then the same becomes a habit. Once you are habituated to discharge your duties with positive thoughts, the influence of all stored negative thoughts become insignificant.

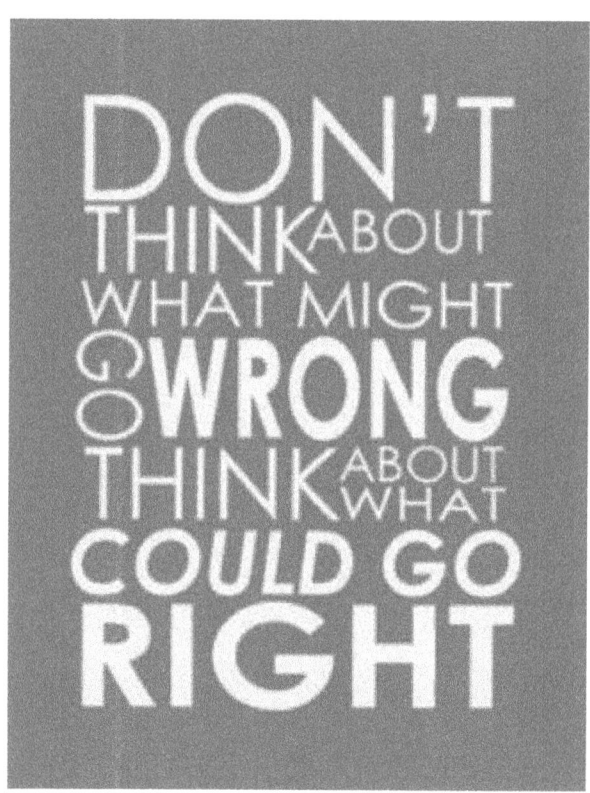

CHAPTER 1

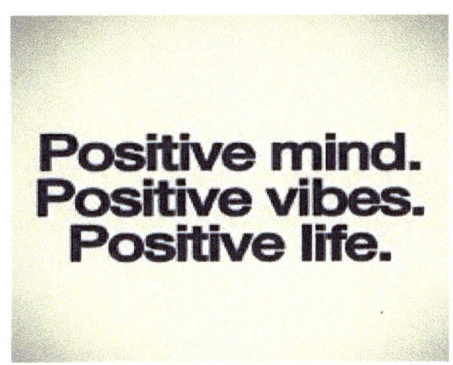

WHAT IS POSITIVE THINKING

The term positive thinking first came into public usage by a christian preacher by the name of norman vincent peale, who wrote a book called the power of positive thinking. The phrase has been hijacked since then by numerous people, mostly in the self help industry, and has a very different meaning today. Peale used the term positive thinking in a very healthy and loving way.

It was mainly around how he believed we should see ourselves as people, and how much we should let god into our lives as a source of strength who could help us change and achieve things that would be truly remarkable. Peale encouraged and believed in a very healthy and strong self image, bolstered by the power of god within us. The modern use of positive thinking virtually always leaves out any sense of god or a higher power and focuses exclusively on a strictly judgmental definition of beliefs and views as being either positive i.e good or negative, ie bad.

So positive thinking is to be happy and grateful and outgoing, and negative thinking is to be unhappy, ungrateful, sorry for yourself etc. That then defines your emotional map, that you need to change from a negative thinking to positive thinking.

Unfortunately this is based on a totally false premise and thus, all that happens is that people effectively go into a state of denial about hoe they feel and just tell themselves that they feel some thing else, that they don't really, and just suppress their true feelings. This can lead to horrific problems both in childhood and further down the line and blocks any really true sense and acceptance of who you are as a person. Its also a million miles from what norman vincent peale actually meant.

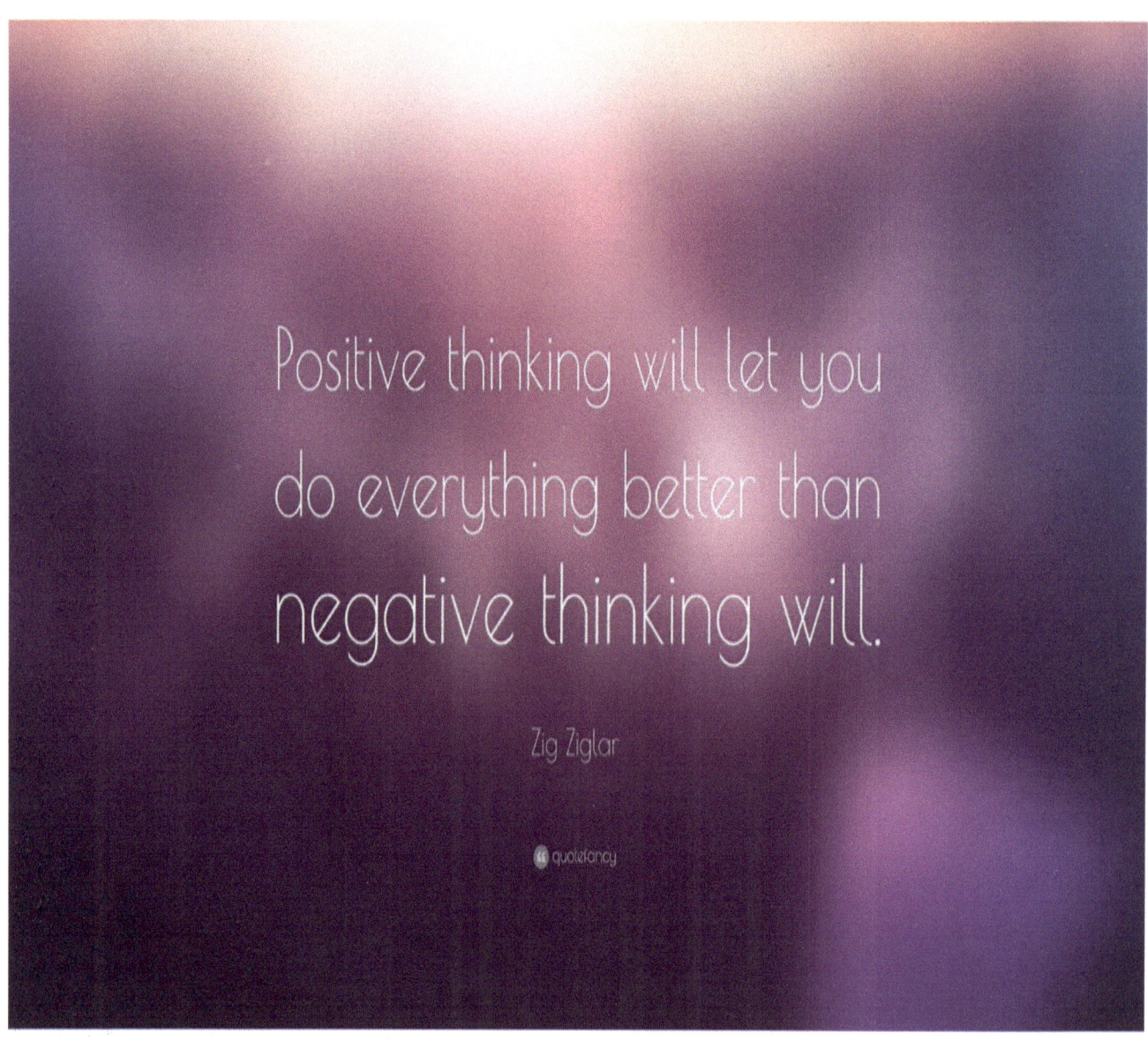

CHAPTER 2

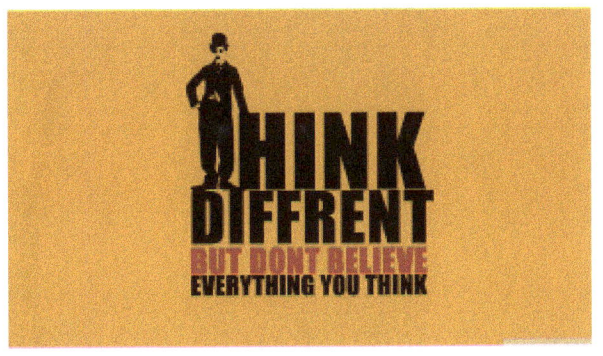

BENEFITS OF POSITIVE THINKING

Positive thinking does create positive outcomes. But not everyone believes that. Some people think positive outcomes are only dictated based on how much effort you put into something. And, while effort counts, how great of an outcome can you have if you think miserably along the journey to that outcome? Some people think positive thinking is a "trendy thing" and that the truth is, "whatever is meant to be will be." And while destiny, fate, etc. can be something to believe in, you must realize that your mind and the energy you give off impacts that destiny. And then, you just have cynical people that always find the bad in situations or play devil's advocate way too much. Well, that is their prerogative, don't feed into it and stay away from them.

If you want more positive outcomes in your life, you do have to think positive. Positive thinking steers your course into a positive outcome. Here are ways positive thinking leads you toward a positive outcome:

1. Positive Thinking Builds Confidence.

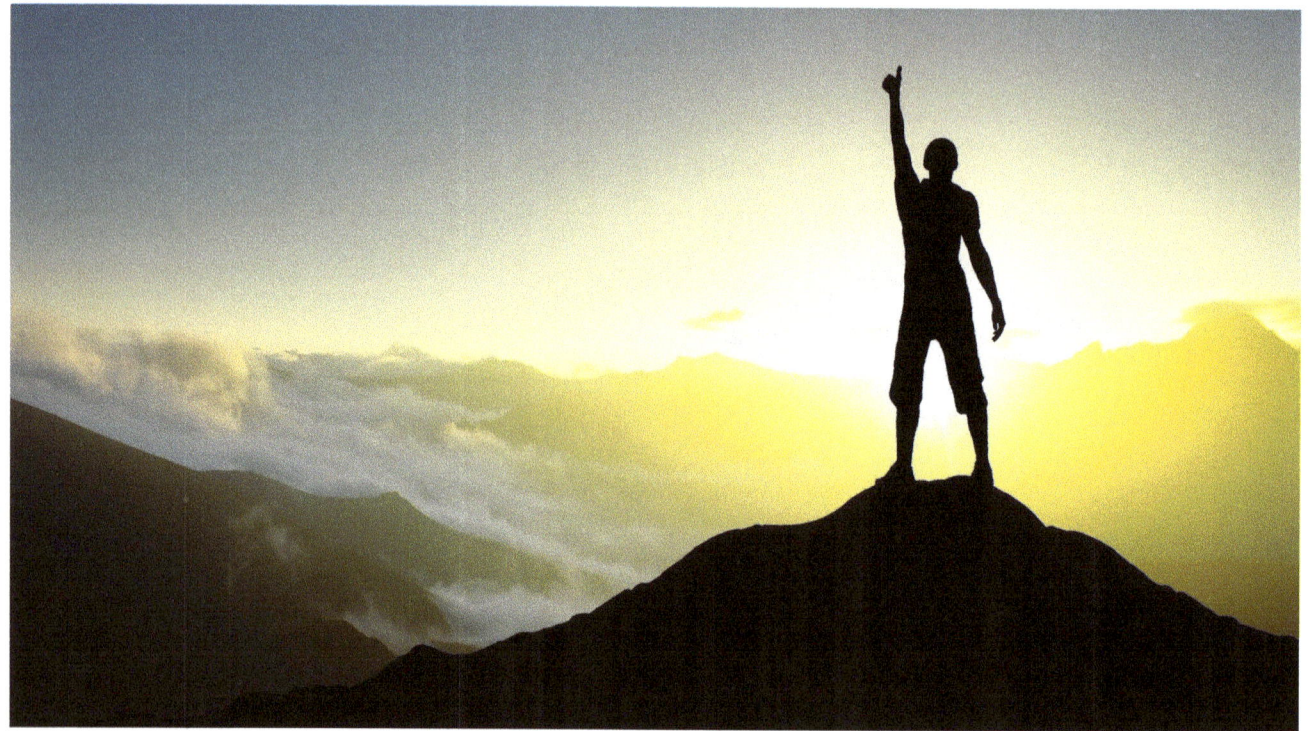

When you think positively you think positive about what is around you. You see the good in life and in people. You trust in yourself and your resources. This process builds confidence. As you see the strength and goodness of your world and yourself, you are more apt to take healthy risks. Instead of letting fear stop you from huge dreams and goals, you are able to believe in yourself and take leaps toward goals. You know that if you hit a barrier, you can hurdle it or those around you will help you hurdle it, and that builds confidence. Confidence is what you need to take risks and risks often lead to positive outcomes, like success.

2. Positive Thinking makes you See More Resources.

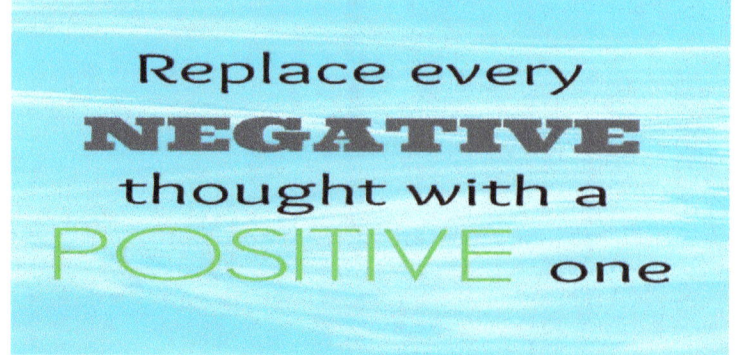

Happy and positive people see what they do have, and that goes for their resources, too. Those who think limitedly, are cynical or fail to see the positive in situations often miss resources that are right around them. They often close their mind to their community and those around them who want to help. You may often hear them use the statement "I always do everything myself." This is a very powerful black and white comment. This type of thinking shuts down a lot of amazingness right around them. Instead, the positive minded person looks at the resources they do have even if they are limited. They will work harder to find resources in the community that could support them. Resources will help you gain momentum, stay your course, and help you hurdle barriers. All things that will lead to a positive outcome.

3. Positive Thinking Keeps You Open-Minded.

Positive people have open minds. They listen to others, not just give their two cents. This gives insight into what people desire, what questions they should ask and alternate points of view. They try to see life through different perspectives. By opening your mind, you see more answers, opportunities and ways to live your life fully. More opportunities, more insights and more fulfillment create more positive outcomes.

4. POSITIVE THINKING CREATES A "SMARTER" BRAIN

Positive thinking also has a positive impact on how the brain itself functions. Research in the field of positive psychology has shown that when a brain is kept positive by maintaining positive attitude, it actually creates more neural pathways faster and has an increased ability to problem solve and "think better." In other words, practicing the power of positive thinking and maintaining positive attitude are like feeding your brain "super food" to help it thrive.

5. The People Around you Will be More Positive

It is no secret that when you are a positive person it will rub off on the people around you. Either they will become more positive or they will tend to fall out of your life to be replaced by people who have a more positive attitude. People with a positive attitude tend to attract other people with positive attitudes. You will find you are much happier if you are surrounded by positive people.

6. People Will Like you Better

When you have a positive attitude people will have a better opinion of you. Not only does this mean that you will have more friends but it will also help you at work. You will find that if you have a positive attitude you will be more likely to be promoted. This goes back to good things happening to people who are able to stay positive.

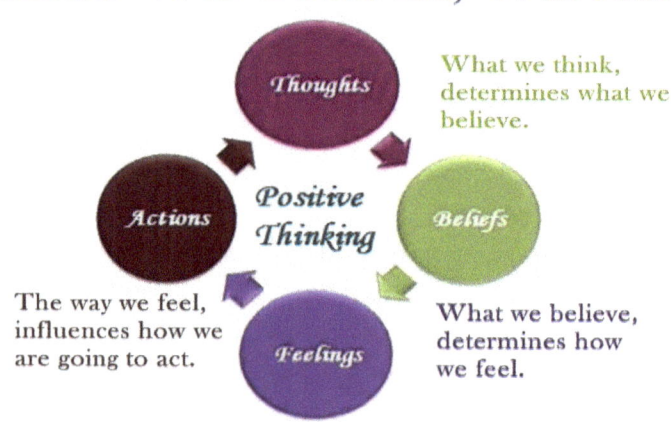

CHAPTER 3

10 RULES OF THE POWER OF POSITIVE THINKING

The power of positive thinking and the top ten rules in getting it is one of the hottest topic today.

This is because people are realizing that positive thinking and a positive attitude does affect life significantly. Have you heard of "The Secret" movie? It's rapidly making it's way around the world.

Whether you see a glass as half-empty or half-full can affect the way you treat yourself. We are in control of our lives and our destiny.

An idle brain, is a devils' workshop they say. This is not a positive quote. However, using this ideology in mind, we ventured to write on positive thinking, so that something productive would be achieved of our minds.

Here are the top **10 Rules to Get the Power of Positive Thinking.**

1) **Believe** - You need to believe. You can not pretend to be a positive thinker. In positive thinking, you can not fake it because there is no one to pretend to. If somebody merely believes that you are a positive thinker, how can that benefit you? The most important of the ten rules of the power of positive thinking is that you yourself should believe it.

2) **Be objective** - This is very important in the ten rules for the power of positive thinking. Many people tend to see their lives for their failures and thus, they lose all hope of ever attaining in their goal. Some other people, filled with false pride, tend to magnify their success and they make all the wrong decisions.

3) **Surround yourself with people who have a positive attitude** - When you are engaged in an internal battle between your negative and positive self, you will need all the help you can get. Do not surround yourself with negative people who will just drag your positive attitude to the floor with their negativity.

4) **Be healthy** - All of the positive thinking in the world will not help you if you are six feet under, can it? You have to keep your body healthy in order to fuel your positive thinking. One step to achieving the power of positive thinking is looking after your body.

5) **Switch negativity around** - Remove all negative thoughts by repelling it outright when something negative enters your personality. Channel that energy into positive thoughts. Positive quotes and positive affirmations will help to keep negativity away.

6) **Be patient** - Positive thinking is not immediate. You need to reprogram yourself in order to get remove any negative attitude you possess.

7) **Remember that other people can sense your negativity** -

Before you do anything, be sure to have the right attitude. One reason why people fail is because others can sense their negative attitude and want no part of it. Positive thoughts, positive thinking, and positive affirmation create a positive attitude

8) **Be positive** - Always look for something positive in everything new. When you encounter something unfamiliar, do not be afraid. Take a hard look at it and see it for the positive effects it brings, this will make your life easier.

9) **Pace yourself** - You need to pace yourself in order to prevent yourself from collapsing. Take life one day at a time. Remember that you can not hurry into being positive. Be patient and you will achieve a positive attitude.

10) **Apply the change** - The main characteristic of these ten rules of the power of positive thinking is the fact that they only bring you to the door. You have to open it yourself. Many individuals do not realize this, but we need these rules in order to appreciate life more. Some people think rules limit our achievements, but this is untrue. Without any rules, we would have been extinct centuries ago. Rules remove the chaos that is called life and impose sanity into it.

Rules are what we use to help us understand the true meaning of life. Sometimes, we look for rules in order to help us attain our goals. People make rules in order to help themselves achieve their goals in a manner that they can understand. Rules are also used to help us understand life. People give out rules in order to help others get what they want. We are able to keep every discovery made because of rules.

It seems that people, when looking for rules, like to stick to ten, which is a nice, round number. It comes as no surprise that individuals look for 10 rules for the power of positive thinking.

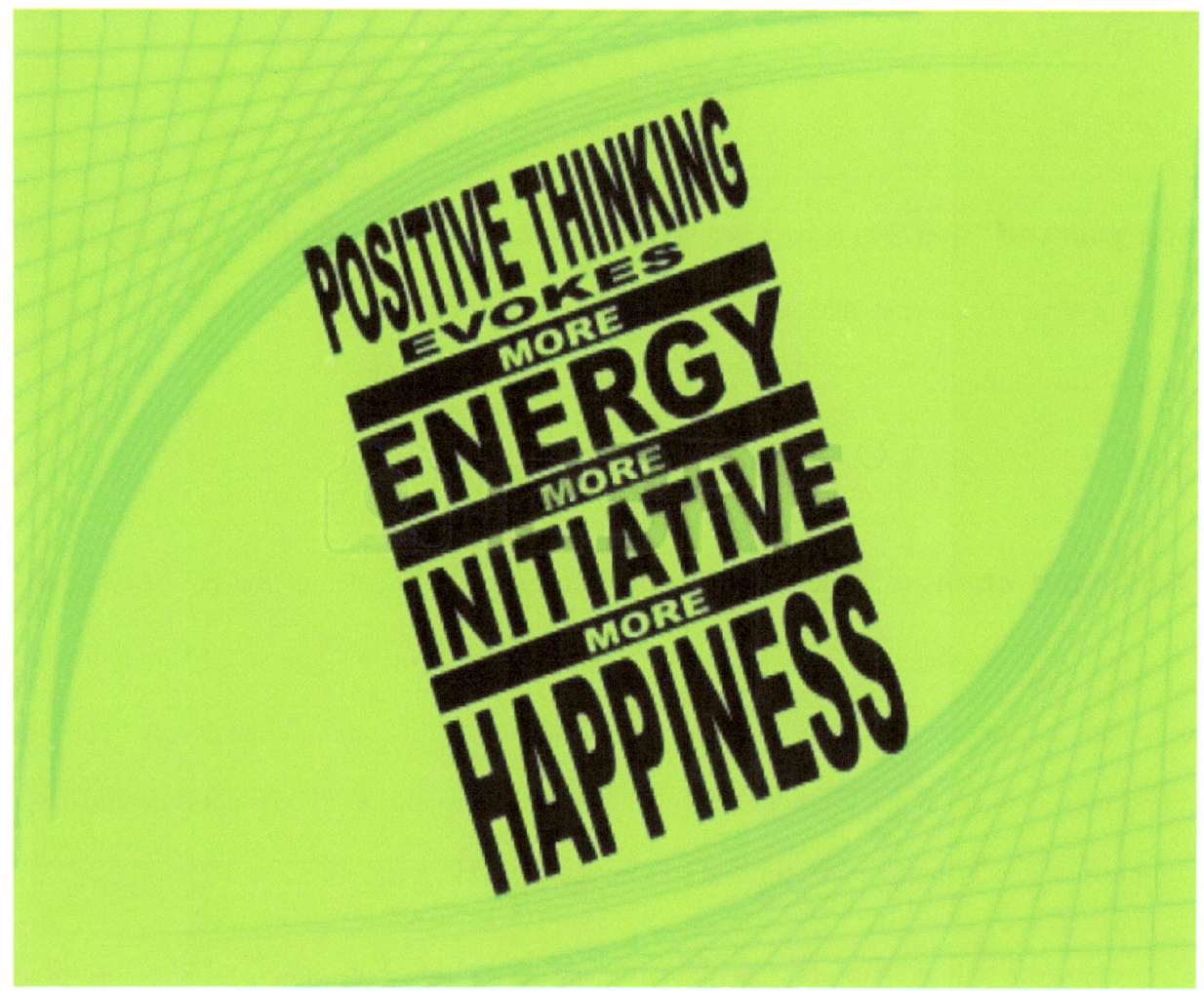

CHAPTER 4

PRACTICAL TIPS FOR POSITIVE THINKING - POSITIVITY CAN BE LEARNED

Why Positivity Can Be Learned.

Wouldn't it be nice to always - or mostly - have positive thoughts?

We have to live inside our heads a large part of our waking life. Granted, when we are working, playing, exercising, or socializing in any way -- relating to family, friends, co-workers, etc...we are taken outside of ourselves, out of our heads, and our own mind-chatter is less present. And these activities are a great way to reduce our mind-chatter when we are feeling negative, and they can lead to a total turn-around too.

But when we are on our own we mostly live inside out heads. And often the inner life in there is not all pleasant. We spend a lot of time in anger, anxiety, strife, worry, fear, negativity, arguments, sadness, brooding, drama, etc...

Instead, we could be planning, dreaming, thinking creative thoughts, having realizations, insights, and breakthroughs, having thoughts of gratitude, enjoyment, fun. We could be experiencing the moment in awe, wonder, enthusiasm, excitement, and feeling waves of passion, ecstasy, and bliss. Yes, these are all valid ways of being, these are all attainable inner states.

Beautifying Your Inner Landscape.

How do we attain such beautiful inner landscapes? Like outer landscapes, they can be cultivated. Some landscapes are born beautiful. Others need a little cultivation.

How Do We Cultivate a Positive Inner Terrain.

How do we cultivate a positive inner terrain? Well, the first and last thing I'm going to tell you is that it comes down to "faith". But I'll tell you a lot of other things in between that can also help you to think positively, and that will also help to build your faith in life.

Positive Thinking is just a Habit.

Positive Thinking is just a habit. It is not rocket science. It is not mumbo jumbo. It is not magic, spiritual, religious or anti-religious. It is simply a habit, that anyone can cultivate. We are all thinking all the time. It might as well be a positive experience!

The Inner Terrain of the Mind.

We are all creatures of habit. Our brain is made up of synapses that are formed through our activities. The more we do something, the stronger the synapse becomes, allowing us to do it better, easier, more often, and with more enjoyment. This creates a habit. When we take conscious steps to break a habit, and we stop the actions, the synapses slowly dissolve and the habit is broken.

How to Cultivate New Habits.

The doing of the habit, the action itself, is the strongest thing we can do in creating a new habit. Thinking about changing our habit, planning to change it, reading about how to change it -- these can all be helpful, but nowhere near as powerful to make real changes as actually doing the habit we want to start. (Or not doing the habit we want to quit).

This is a terrifically important thing to understand on a deep level. If you want to think positively, start thinking positive thoughts. Think one right now. "I am OK". (for instance)..

Journal Exercise - Developing A New Synapses

Fill in the blank with the best believable thing you can think about yourself: "I am _____".

Or, if you can't think something positive about yourself just yet, start with thinking something positive about someone else. "Jim is OK". "Mom is doing great". "Carrie is a wonderful friend". Now its your turn:

"_____ is _____"

Now, you've established a new synapses in your brain's inner-talk landscape. You'll strengthen this synapses with repetition throughout the day of similar positive thoughts. You'll add many more soon.

I want you to write down as many positive thoughts as you can. Don't worry about whether or not they feel true to you just yet. If you write them now, at some point they will pop back in to your head as genuine positive thoughts.

Here are some of my positive thoughts that I seem to be able to dredge up even in the darkest times...

I am good

I am full of love

I want the best for all people

I love my children/ family

I am grateful for my health

Now, write down in your journal as many positive thoughts as you can...

Negative Thinking is Just a Habit

Negative thinking is just a habit! It is not who you are. It is not a reflection of any defect in you. It is simply a habit.

Our brain is a chemical factory manufacturing our emotions. When we feel a certain emotion a lot, our brain manufactures a lot of the chemical that communicates that emotion to your body. When that chemical floods your body and is picked up at receptor sites, a lot, then the body produces more receptors for that chemical. This creates a chemical addiction to that emotion.

To start out with in life, 90% of our receptor cells are joy receptors. We are coded for joy.

Like synapses, receptors increase with use, and dissolve with lack of use.

Habits take 21 days to create.

For 21 days, come up with your own joy-enhancing program including positive thinking. Or follow mine below.

Here is my idea of a 21-day-positive-program:

My 21-Days to Positivity Program

For 21 Days...

- Do something you love each day.

- Make a list of positive thoughts each morning.

- Start the day doing the thing you love best for an hour.

- Exercise for an hour each day.

- Eat a big salad each day.

- Have some fruit each day.

- Spend some time alone in thought, contemplation, meditation, or prayer each day.

- End each day with a list of things you are grateful for.

You can alter it for your lifestyle preferences, your unique personality, and your beliefs. Be creative.

Pitfalls to Positive Thoughts

Some things to watch out for...

Here are some long-term habits that can sabotage positive thinking:

- over-use of sarcasm or cynicism

We might think we're being witty, but the sarcastic or cynical attitude is addictive and can derail positive thinking. Some people are more cynical than others, and that might be your nature. I think you can find a balance in which you can be yourself and still enjoy your thought-life. A sense of humor is very helpful to this personality type.

- criticism of others

We might spend a lot of time thinking about the flaws of others. This can be highly habit forming, consuming many a life. Maybe this keeps our mind off our own problems. Often it is a way to avoid facing our own issues. It is however not conducive to positive thinking. Criticizing or blaming others keeps us stuck and keeps us from growing through actually facing our own issues.

- self-criticism

We can get really caught up in thinking about our own flaws, problems, and issues. Through our habit-forming brain and its synapses and our habit-forming body and its receptors for emotion-chemicals, we can turn this self-criticism in to a depressing habit. Start finding and creating the good in yourself!

- doubt

I think humans have a lot of faith naturally, in each other, in themselves, in this place we live in called reality, the world, or The Universe. Babies and small children have this kind of total faith. Bad experiences can cause us to start doubting ourselves and others. This is where faith becomes a necessity to keep us from this positivity-draining emotion of doubt.

- blame

A lot of us form the habit of blaming others. This is a nice way to avoid dealing with our own problems. But the mind-chatter of blaming covers up any possibility of positive thinking the same way pollution covers up the blue sky. Blaming also keeps us from growing. You can stagnate for years with this mechanism.

- guilt and shame

Feeling ashamed or guilty as a long-term habitual mind-set gets your energy so far down that positive thinking can be quite elusive. A little guilt or shame can be a good catalyst for change. But hanging on to an emotion like this as a long-term habit can't be very helpful. Lighten up on yourself. Let it go.

Practices that lead to Positive Thinking

1. A Good Start:

Start each day off with positive thinking, through a prayer of gratitude, meditation, journaling, or making a list of things your are thankful for.

2. Affirmations:

You don't have to do these now, but whenever you choose. It could be when you need to drum up some positive thoughts. Or it could be when you are feeling really happy and want to capture and expand this feeling in to more of your life!

Make a list of positive affirmations, things you like about yourself, your immediate family members, and others you interact with regularly.

Make a list of things affirming your faith in the Universe...I am loved, My greatest good along with the greatest good of all is always being met, everything works together for the good, there are not very many real emergencies, etc...

Make a list of affirmations of things you love....I love life, I love people, I love my family, etc...

Make a list of things you enjoy....I enjoy going out with a good friend, I enjoy walks in nature, I enjoy playing with my kids, etc....

Make a list of things you want. Now make a list converting each of these things in to an affirmation, as though you already have it, or its already on its way.

These are all the types of things we think about, and by doing affirmations on paper, you are programming your brain to actually start thinking about things in a positive light.

3. Discipline:

"You can not afford the luxury of a negative thought". Since thoughts are habits, one negative one can snowball in to a totally negative mind-state. If you know the thoughts that set you off, you can banish them the moment they set in. I tell myself, I feel pretty good right now, and I deserve to keep feeling good, so I would rather not think that thought. Sometimes it doesn't go away right away, but I just don't give it any energy, and so it goes eventually.

You know the old Indian story about the Grandfather who tells his Grandson about a battle going on inside him between two wolves, one who is greedy, frightened, and angry, and one who is kind, peaceful, and loving. "Which one will win?" asks the Grandson. And his Grandfather answers: "The one I feed".

4. Prayer:

You can not be too negative when you are talking to the Creator of the Universes. It tends to bring out the best in us. And positive mind-states will come upon us sooner or later as a result of prayer.

5. Meditation:

Sitting or lying and focusing on our breathing for 5-15 minutes, or longer, we can just watch our thoughts and observe them without judging them. It is as though we are a third party outside of our mind, just noticing what is going on there.

6. Doing What We Love:

Doing what we love will make us happy, and when we're happy our thoughts are positive. If possible, make a career of the thing you love doing. Otherwise, spend an hour a day doing what you love, -

ideally the first hour. You'll find yourself thinking more positively automatically.

7. Loving What We Do:

When we put our full attention and effort on something, we can't help but love it. So, whatever we find ourselves doing in life, do it without fear, and with all the caring we can muster. Positive thoughts will automatically follow.

8. Faith, The Final Frontier:

After practicing all kinds of things for positive thinking, I wound up realizing that my missing link was faith. I realized that I had stopped having faith. I don't know when it happened. I'm all for personal religious experience vs. church, but I guess one of the risks of being away from association with other religionists is that you can forget your faith. I was still praying. Still giving thanks. But I had purposely thrown myself in to matters of material living because I have a tendency to keep my head in the clouds otherwise.

For a while I was so worried about business it was starting to affect my health and sanity. One day during this long period of struggle and strife I suddenly realized that I was not having faith. The idea hit me like a ton of bricks. Wow, I can't believe that I forgot to have faith!

And suddenly my faith came pouring back in to me. Of course everything is going to be OK. Of course everything is happening in perfect divine order. And of course there is nothing to fear. I am taken care of, I am loved, I am receiving exactly the lessons I need, there is nothing I can't handle, I am part of the divine plan in which the greatest good of all beings is being taken in to consideration.

And by thinking these types of thoughts we activate something that makes it so.

I think that I had faith before, but not "living faith". "Faith" can be a noun, something that you possess. But "living faith" is active, a verb.

I am of no particular religious persuasion. But I am interested in all religions. I think that no matter what religious or spiritual practices we have, that we can all access faith. We can all believe in a higher power or our own higher power. This is faith. Knowing that it is not just us in control of our life. That we can ask for help, that we can receive help, that we are loved and cared for, that the Universe is on our side. And being open to this help, this love. And trusting it.

I think most people have had an experience of a benevolent "presence". Or they have had fleeting glimpses of some power outside of themselves helping and affecting their lives.

If not a "believer" in a higher power outside of ourselves, perhaps one could imagine a Unified Consciousness, in which all humans are joined as One. This Consciousness could be made of Love, and one could have faith in this greater Oneness of humanity.

CONCLUSION

POSITIVE THINKING: THE ESSENCE OF EXISTENCE

Positive thinking is a vibe that could easily fool the heart. At adverse times, when one thinks positive thoughts and acts on them, the mind could be controlled to relax and help see the big picture. People always assume that only the ones who are logical and have a practical or realistic approach to life succeed. But, that is not entirely true. Being logical or practical or realistic is important to succeed but staying positive and focused in equally important. A person with positive attitude and thoughts is said to have won half the battle even before it has begun.

This is clearly illustrated in the fact that Late Mr. Steve Jobs, who is the pillar behind Apple Inc. was at one point fired from his own company by a fellow colleague who he hired. But, he was not bogged down by this incident. Rather he was determined to take over the company again. He succeeded in becoming the CEO of Apple Inc. in a few years time and continued to be in the same position till his death recently. It was positive thinking with hard work and determination that helped him make Apple Inc. the company it is today. If Jobs had given way to negative thoughts we would have not seen the iPod and IPhone that are famous today.

Negativity in life drains out all the good things about a man. Positivity can change the life you are living and help you create your future that is more fulfilling and worth living. Everyone has a dream that is not lived because of the negative influence from people around us or taught by them. The worst of all is; most of the time people fail in life because they do not have the courage to live their dream fearing failure. One should build up an attitude that gives the perspective to look at failures as positive steps towards success. One should take measures to train the brain to look at failures as positive points that make them strong.

J.K. Rowling, the author of Harry Potter series of books did not turn rich overnight. She had to face 15 rejections of the first book before she was accepted to be published. She was a then recently divorced single mother who had no job and left without a penny. She had enough reasons to be a failure, but it was positive thinking and the ability to see the bigger picture in spite of the obstacle that has made her richer than the Queen of England.

Our brain is designed to give instructions on our day to day activities. It is our thought processes that have derived the formula and instructed the brain to dictate the actions. We are masters and we can always change the rules and ignore the nagging negative voice that has been put there by us over years of time. But, positive attitude is not something one can gain immediately. Negativity and pessimism are more like a disease that has to be cured over a period of time with effective training. Failures and negative feedbacks did not stop Thomas Edison from inventing many things which include the Light Bulb. He faced more than 1000 failures before he successful lit a bulb.

To develop positive thinking one must always make conscious choices and decisions and never allow pre determined thoughts take the action course. The decision that one takes must focus only on the bigger picture. The mind is trained to believe certain things and ignore certain things as 'too good to be true'. Stephenie Meyer, a novelist who is famous for the Twilight series of books refused to publish them when friends asked her to do so because the story was good. Only after persuasion from a close friend she sent it to 15 literary houses to be ignored by 9 and rejected by 5. One agreed to publish and today she is reported to have made $40 million from this book series alone. It is true that if people around us can impact our thoughts and life in a negative way, they can do the same in a positive way too. Try and stay away from people who say you can't.

Seeing a bigger picture and creating a better future for yourself is difficult but not impossible. The secret recipe is, positive thinking.

Here are the four golden rules that you should remember day in and day out:

- Acknowledge the fact that you are a person with negative thinking and ready to change.

- Ignore all negative thoughts coming from within and negative words coming from people around you. Convert them as motivation factors and work on proving them wrong.

- There is no such thing as predetermined fate. Your fate and future is what you make or break.

- Nurture the creativeness from within and utilize the opportunities provided or create your own opportunities.

When building a positive mentality, you will face hurdles that you might and might not have control over. You should be aware of them and be ready to face them when you stumble upon them. Positive thinking will help you be successful not only in your professional life but also in your personal life because both go hand in hand. Most people fail in personal life because they failed in professional life and vice versa. But, that is not applicable to people who are believers. With positive thinking, you might not become a millionaire over night but, you will be happy and satisfied with what you have at the end of the day.

Being positive and have an open mind towards life is a wisdom gained through hard work and go a long way. But, once you master the technique of positive thinking, you can be happy and self sufficient even with a dollar in your pocket. Said and done, positive thinking never lets you down even if friends and family do in the hour of need. Give in yourself to positive thinking and you can live your life everyday unlike the people who die every day.

7 RULES OF LIFE

1. Make peace with your past so it does not affect the present.

2. What others think of you is none of your business.

3. Time heals almost everything, give it time.

4. Don't compare your life to others and don't judge them. You have no idea what their journey is all about.

5. It's alright not to know all the answers. They will come to you when you least expect it.

6. You are in charge of your happiness.

7. Smile. You don't own all the problems in the world.

www.ingramcontent.com/pod-product-compliance
Lightning Source LLC
Chambersburg PA
CBHW061148010526
44118CB00026B/2905